I0776575

<u>Dedicated To My Parents</u>

I never needed to refer autobiography of any successful people, because synonym of success for me is you, mom-dad….

I never needed sympathy and help of any one because my strongest backbone is you, mom-dad…..

I never needed to go temple and praying for my desire because who fulfilled my untold wishes is you, mom-dad…..

I never needed to give up in life because the reason behind my winning attitude is you, mom-dad…

Introduction

One year after my daughter's birth, I got some "me" time and I sat down to gather my thoughts on my experience of motherhood. I paused staring picture of my childhood and went into the flashback. Writing has been my passion, since I was a teenager. Right from my school days, I would pen down everything that crossed my mind. I was a bright student. I was more interested in elocution competitions and assay writings than sports. My parents were teachers. So, I got advantage of reading lots of books of their libraries during vacations. I would sit by the balcony side of my home and could read whole book in one sitting without eating and drinking.

As time passed, I started giving less time to my writing and reading passion as I wanted to become a doctor. I had to study, give exams and to attend so many other competitions so life started to get busy. Then I never got enough time to sit with myself. As I grew, I never got enough time for writing except some poems.

I am M.Pharm by profession and started working as an Assistant Professor at Pharmacy College. Journey had been not at all so smooth so far. But, I was very positive and full of life. I was always trying to be happy in any worst condition. And then, like with many Indian moms, there comes a time when my mom felt, I should marry. I was ambitious independent girl and was not ready for marriage. But its "SOCHA NA THA" movie type love story so after dating I find the love of my life and I got married and thoroughly enjoyed this phase of life. After marriage, I continued to work. I am lucky to get husband cum friend. After three years of marriage, I blessed with the most beautiful angel sent from God that filled my life with joy, love and gave an entire new meaning to my journey. I became a mother of charming daughter and motherhood gave new meaning to my life. With my baby's birth, a mother was born too. I cannot forget ever, how life drastically changed 180 degrees after that first crying of her than ever but of course they are and will the happiest times of my life. I have always been a working woman and suddenly after the baby, like many other moms, I left my job and decided to take a long break.

Motherhood brings unconditional joy and love to my life but I believe it's equally very important to remember our own identity and never stop doing what we love. When I looked at my husband, he still continued to do everything he did before becoming a father. From an assistant professor to full time house wife and baby sitting definitely a big change in my life. When this happened, I didn't understand how to keep myself creatively occupied. I didn't ready to send my daughter in any day care and I had not trust on any nanny (obviously there are lots of good day care and nanny but it's my choice). Then I decide to do something by staying at home. I started my online business to sell stuff but there was something that I was still missing. One day I was feeling tired and frustrated so my husband suggests me that I should write a book about my experiences of motherhood. If I want to write, then he would help me. Well, that was no less than a "aha" moment for me that changed my life instantly. I am also online tutor, but only my passion for writing relishes me. It was like, I could put my heart out to likeminded people in the world. I could never imagine connecting with people across the world to being an author. I decided to write a book on motherhood not only to write my mind and share my views but also to help new moms and mom to be to that how to mentally and emotionally prepare yourself for this monumental experience in your life, how to keep happy with a hundred doubts and insecurities about being able to handle motherhood.

Well, my journey from motherhood to being a writer mommy is adventurous roller coaster ride. I never imagined this could be the power of motherhood and also never felt such things could happen with me. I would like to share my emotional rainbow of motherhood with you. I am sure you will easily connect this with yourself. Finally, to all the new mommies in the house, there can never be anything better than love yourself and do what you want to do because this is the only thing that makes you happy. Cheers for motherhood...!!!

(Note: The views, recommendations and opinions expressed in this book are solely according to my experience and understanding. So please consult your doctor for professional advice concerning specific health/medical matters.)

Acknowledgment

This book is dedicated to my pretty daughter "Pihu" who gives meaning to my life and my parents who are my strongest backbone, who taught me how to live life fearlessly. Of course, this would not have been possible without my best friend and blessings of God- my loving husband "Ankit". I also dedicate this book to parenting site momspresso.com (formerly known as mycity4kids.com) whose articles inspired me a lot. Thanks to God, that I could do this and I feel you are present around me to complete this book.

Index

1.

So, are you going to become mom, huh..??

Pregnancy is one of the most crucial phase of woman's life especially for first time mommy. Till today, I remember the day when those two pink lines on the test kit appeared and report was positive. I was acting like crazy, cranky and funny because of hormonal changes. What a major mood swings I experienced..!!

I could never forget experience of my first labour and nervousness. How I felt my child want to come out in this beautiful earth during diwali time. Hearing the first cry of my kid, I too cried and held my mom and forgot that unforgettable pain while a moment. I didn't wish to know the gender and just asked my mom that "Is my baby ok or not?" My blood group is negative and we were living in small town. It was diwali time and all specialist doctors went on holidays. So, I was worried about my delivery. Life has totally changed after becoming a mom but it also has been the best landmark of my life.

As I look at my little girl play, run and laugh, I go into flashback and remember the magnificent days of my pregnancy. I lived with my husband alone during seven months of pregnancy and we walked this beautiful journey together. We wanted our baby to be born healthy and happy, like any other parents. I think couples that can feel and face a pregnancy as a team, can survive anything together in life. Mood swings aside, I was so suspicious about everything related to the baby's healthy growth too. I was doing just about everything that I possibly could, to make sure I didn't go wrong anywhere with my baby. I never ignored any piece of suggestion; I was always all ears. Whenever I see would-be moms, I always sense their faces overflowing with a mixture of all emotions at this amazing phase of their lives. This looks more noticeable on the faces of first-time moms. Some women experience an easy going pregnancy, while others face some complications but the essence of motherhood has the power to overcome all. Based on my experience, I would like to share few things for first-time moms to make their pregnancy more comfortable:

Enjoy ample amounts of sleep and love yourself:

Love your beautiful body, flat belly and enjoy your peaceful sleep because once baby will come, its gone forever. A healthy body is only possible if you have a happy mind and enough rest. Do away with your worries, in a case of any complexity; your doctor will try his level best to work it out. You will feel fresh if you have a good sleep and that will keep you active and charged for your set of activities.

Healthy Diet:

Pregnancy can be the best experience of a woman's life if it is healthy. My aunt says woman who has craving for sweet give birth to a girl and craving for spicy food leads to a baby boy. This is a pure myth, but during my third trimester I got into crazy sweet cravings. I got crazy for "laddu" and I gave birth to a baby girl. But don't trust on it. Gender can never be decided by your food cravings. It is a funny prediction. I had face problems of nausea and vomiting. I didn't like healthy diet but I knew I had to eat healthy to stay healthy for myself and my baby so I made a health chart for my pregnancy. I loved to drink coconut during pregnancy. Sometimes I got into badly 'panipuri' and 'chaat' cravings. Sometimes it's ok to eat street food but always remember whatever you eat must be hygienic. A healthy pregnancy means a healthy baby, so prepare diet chart for you after consulting your doctor and try to provide all adequate nutrition to your baby in the womb especially if you are vegetarian like me.

The Weight Phobia- Take it easy:

Many women worry a lot about their weight during pregnancy. I did too. I have always been slim and after my first trimester I was growing fat from size zero. It's going to happen, and you need to let it happen. Stop looking at your body but start to talk with your tummy. I had learnt that the babies gain majority of their strength and nutrition in the womb. You should stop counting your calories and worry about every pound. You are absolutely not going to remain fatty after your baby will born. And putting on weight does not necessarily mean you will not be able to lose it later on. You sure will. You need not eat everything you see but be smart in choosing diet plan.

Google   is   not   Gynaecologist:
The minute most women discover that they are

pregnant; they get into an overdrive of trying to get as much information as possible on what to do and not to do in the months ahead. We are curious to know every small piece of our pregnancy but there are high chances to come across scary stories and wrong information. In the case of doubts arising in your mind, it's always better to consult your doctor. You can also refer parenting sites but don't blindly trust it. Every pregnancy is different from the other. Don't read or browse about some symptoms related to pregnancy which you are also experiencing as it would lead to more panic. I became cranky and scary after reading many articles and consult my doctor for any silly matters. I think he needs a pat on his back for answering all my stupid questions with smile.

Always remember "law of attraction":

Your mental state of happiness will help you deal with your pregnancy with ease. The secret of happiness is to celebrate womanhood and share a healthy loving relationship with your child, it's essential to feel love with yourself. If you over think about any matter, your mind invites negative thoughts indirectly. Remember that whatever you think either positive or negative that comes to you according to law of attraction. So be comfortable with yourself and accept your hormonal changes. Stay positive and follow a healthy routine and be a part of a happy environment, stay away from negativities and feel you are an iron lady who is going to be super woman as a Mom.

The flow of advices and burden of suggestions:

Your pregnancy is a thrilled affair for your immediate family and extended family. Always ready to hear suggestions and advices pouring for you from your well wishers but take it easy. Before doing anything according to anyone's advice, be sure about whether you are comfortable doing it or not. Embrace your inner mom-rebel and say good bye to advice that is not right for you.

Make memories and do mental makeup:

Memory is a way of holding onto the things you love and never want to lose….This is the most memorable phase of your life. You want the phase to get over as soon as possible, but one day you will look back at this time and would want to and rush back those memories over and over again (especially when you are not planning for second child). So take photos of you every month. Start to pen down your experiences and feelings. Do something memorable on your baby shower and click lots of photos with baby bump. Also mentally prepare yourself for your upcoming 24*7 job without leaves. Parenthood is a lifetime responsibility. Being an irresponsible parent is worst thing than anything else. So plan for it mentally, physically and financially.

Trust me; this is the most beautiful phase to love yourself and womanhood. Follow your heart, be yourself and don't worry about standards of perfection laid down by others. Motherhood made me laugh, made me cry and brought out this old passion of writing in me that I never knew even possible. So try to enjoy this phase as much as possible. Take care would be moms….

2.

My First Letter to My Baby!

My little heart, Chiku! This is your secret name that me and your papa have been always calling you, since the time we knew you started your journey in my tummy. You are our first child, and to be honest, we had no idea what we were doing. I had to learn it all with you. I saw you first time when you were around 5 weeks and looking like little egg. And that was the moment I realized that I was going to nurture beautiful life inside me and I thanked god to blessed me with pregnancy.

I was full of excitement. I didn't understand what to do. I called your maasi and start to crying and then laughing. I felt that I was going to became mad soon, due to rainbow of emotions inside me. I couldn't wait to be your mamma. I have studied everything I could about how to be a good mom, how to help you learn and grow and how to be the best example I can be for you.

Your papa also gifted me book of "Garbh Sanskar". When I was choosing a husband, I decided to choose the man with the biggest most beautiful heart and family values, I could find and that's your papa. I and your papa were very excited when my doctor put the foetal doppler and we first time heard your heart beat. When you were of 13 weeks I and papa could see your arms and legs shaping up in the hospital scanning room and doctor said that your child was looking very naughty. Your baby was doing yoga in belly; since that day, I wanted to see you more and more, every day! I and papa were so silly that we discussed about purchasing sonography machine. So, we can see you and feel you whenever we want.

Sometimes I had the childish idea of taking you out; hold you in my arms; taking with you;

sleeping with you; giving you lots of kisses and hugs and then putting you back into my tummy. I always asked you what you want to eat. I was super excited to see you again at 29 weeks along with your granny! Every month with my growing belly I could feel you and that makes me proud of being into motherhood. I relish every bit of your kicks, rolling over and stretches. I am not worried about my stretch marks, because I knew it's a good sign that you were growing inside me!

Sometimes I wanted to scold you due to your kicks in tummy, when I was taking lecture at college. Students were looked at me and give smile to each other. Sometimes I used to feel nervous whenever there was constant vomiting, stomach pain and no movement...maybe you were sleeping along with me. Your tiny presence made me strong to come over my emotional breakdowns and mood swings.

Your mamma is carrier oriented and always likes to be a working mom but you are always and will be my first priority. I will never let you alone. This day you were of 36 weeks and I was waiting to hold you in my arms, hug you, see your smile, play with you, kiss you and introduce you to this beautiful world. I wish that your first day on earth would be on "Dhanteras-A very precious day in India in Hindu Religion" but it was your choice. I don't know when you will be able to read and really understand this. But always remember, I will always love you the most and I will always be available on every front of your life to guide you any time. I promise to make your every birthday special and different. I promise to build one library for you at home. I will help you learn to read and then I will share you all the stories that your granny told me. As a mom, I would like to pass on some lessons from my experiences, which I learnt in my life.

You are lucky that your papa is fond of movies. He told me to build home theatre for you at home. He is excited to watch harry porter, home alone and baby's day out, and lots of cartoon movies with you. I promise you are girl or boy we will give you equal importance and freedom to live your life on your way. We never pass on our dreams on you, but help you to fulfil your dreams and always remember you are my life and me and papa always loves you. I hope you will love to sleep like me and also allowed me to sleep. Ha ha…! Whole country is busy and excited to celebrate Diwali and New Year. But I am eagerly waiting for you my little cracker. Come soon... Mamma wants to celebrate Diwali with you. Love you already! Mommy

3.

We made some rules that we never follow!!!

We made instruction manual for us during my pregnancy that what to do and don't do after baby. Here are some rules that we never follow:

No fights in front of the baby

We decided to be a team as a parent. Ha Ha!!!!!! This is never possible for us. Our choices and way of handing our baby was very different. So there were lots of little fights because of our notorious girl. And our little one cheers for that.

Set the routine for the baby

We decided that we try to sleep early and wake up early. No late night outing and movies. But my girl didn't like to sleep at night. So, during weekend we went for late night outing and saw cartoon movies with her.

Become chilled out parents and fulfil all her demands

We decided that we never become hyper and tense about her activity of making home messy: "Oh, my god, How could you do this???" "Why are you painting walls??" "Don't play outside, it`s raining." We wished to gift her all the things she wants but now realized going to shop does not mean buying all the things for her. We have to maintain financial budget for her education and future. It`s not necessary to buy something for her every time and if she does something wrong then it`s ok to scold a little in front of others. Kids should have that fear that everything they do is not acceptable and allowed.

No desserts unless baby eat veggies

I want to dish out lots of fruits and veggies, when she started solids. But as like her papa, she loves desserts. So I give myself permission to have desserts for dinner and get back to pushing green veggies next day.

No mobile and more than one hour of TV per day

Electronic gadget in moderation is not evil incarnate and there are times when it can be absolute handy. On days when my girl was sick or not ate well, I allowed her spend few hours a day watching her favourite cartoon and watching rhymes on you tube. Sometimes it`s critical, when I had to do some important works and my little girl is crying for chocolates. It`s difficult to deal with your colicky baby in nuclear set up when there was no one except me to play with her. Another fact was all parents want perfection in their child. So, whenever she went outside to play, there is no one to play with her. All kids of my apartment doing after school activities.

Never use diaper

Before I became mom, I used to critic moms who used diaper for their kids and assuming that how can a mom for her convenience uses diaper all the time. But when I had a baby, I realized that using a diaper can be useful in avoiding unwanted stress. One month after my baby's birth, winter started and there were bunches of people visiting her. So, she could not get enough sleep at day time. She was feeling sleepy at night but she peed 5 times in one hour. So it was difficult to manage her sleep (of course even mine). Sometimes I forgot to check and she was started becoming cranky and crying loudly because of wetness. This might lead to cold and cough. Sometimes she had pooped and soiled her clothes. After putting her on diaper we were sleep peacefully. So it`s not bad to use diapers according to your convenience. Just you have to choose brand wisely to avoid rashes.

I will get back into shape

This one I made for myself. I decided to do exercise and yoga every day. And stop eating for two. But I didn't need it because my girl is notorious and keep me on my toes. So, get back in shape after one year.

Parenthood is the best blessings from God. So bringing your little munchkin home is a special moment, so it's ok if there are few fights to strictly follow rules that make the memory more special and you are going to laugh over it later. It's a slow learning process. So, do away your worries and go ahead, break the rules and celebrate your baby's home coming.

4.

The day when, with my baby, mom inside me was also born..!!

People say "Life is a Journey". But in reality it is a constant learning curve. During my journey from daughter to mother, I found myself continuously rediscovering myself. Life has never been the same after you see the double pink line in the test strip.

November 9th 2015, a day when I feel the meaning of womanhood. That was the happiest day of my life. I was given half anaesthesia and my lower body was made numb. I could not understand what was happening. Suddenly I heard the voice of my aunt, "little laxmi arrived." I could not believe that I delivered baby normally and now she was out of my womb. It was a day of "Dhanteras-A very precious day in India in Hindu

Religion" There were a whole bunch of family members who were crowded around my baby and said: Finally, God fulfilled your wish... after become conscious I wailed about how I hadn't even had a chance to hold my baby yet and everyone had already started playing and laughing with her. That burst of possessiveness was something I was totally unprepared for. My sister's three years old son was very excited to see little tiny baby and wanted to hug her so I got angry and shouted, "Stay away from her. You might hurt her tiny body". Everybody looked at me and I felt guilty. I didn't understand why I scolded my nephew. My sister smiled at me and said, "Welcome to motherhood". At that time, I realised that mom inside me was also born.

I got a chance to finally hold my little daughter in my arms for the first time and looked at her: pretty eyes and bright face. That moment was priceless. I felt the bliss of motherhood first time. I knew life will not be the same anymore. I smiled, touched her soft cheeks, kissed her and bursting into happy cries. Then I fed her first time with the help of nurse. I could not sleep whole night because of pain and rainbow of emotions. I felt my inner soul asked me "Are you ready for being a mom of daughter?" This question irritated me. Somewhere in my mind, I heard, "No! Not yet." I had read everything I could on being a new mom: books about motherhood, the advice columns, credible mom's articles and mom's blogs. Yet I was confused and scared. My girl was very cute, charming and beautiful and I liked her instantly. But every mom likes her baby. It's not a new thing. I was still confused. I felt something was absent. I was anxious that was I capable to brought up a baby?? The moment was so strange that I could not put that in words. I heard so many things from my friends who are moms about sleepless nights, unending crying, the overwhelming love, the nasty diapers and no personnel life. There have definitely been moments of anxiety and self doubt.

The next day I managed to sit up and hold my baby and I forgot everything I had read. I looked at her and I realised how much I drastically changed after being a mom. Everything has been an adventure but I was learning to settle down, although at a slow pace. The feeling of becoming an anxious and scary mom was slowly settling down. I was slowly leant to give bath and massage to her from my 'malishwali'. I was slowly learnt how to breastfeed her. I was slowly learnt to sing lubberly. I slowly used to feel comfortable with dirty diapers and midnight walking to stop her crying. I was slowly learnt to deal with my little devil with patience. I would always wonder at the fact that how my mum would so easily manage so many things together as a working woman and raised four kids, until I became a mom. Nothing prepared me for the realisation that how the sleepless nights will seem less frustrating when I see a big toothless smile. Most of the times I fully enjoy watching her experiments with stuff around. I loved her company over any number of other activities. And I was so glad that this was something I got to learn too. I felt tantrum of her is less irritating when she puts a bunch of kisses on my cheeks and called me 'meemee'. Whenever I was disturbed and ready to burst and then I see my girl's cute innocent face, the frustration was somehow replaced with bliss to do anything and I forget the depression. I forget my stretch marks and fatty tummy when she enjoyed jumping on it. Her presence makes me stronger as a mom day by day. I have a tiny being who thinks the world of me. She come running to me, no matter what, hold me tight while sleeping, even if she gave me a hard time on full day. The journey of being a mom of a new born to being a mom of an extremely energetic kid has been more fun than anything else I have ever done. It has made me more open to seeing goodness of life and made me optimist. There may be challenges all the way but always remember if there is a will, there is a way. Those sleepless nights were soon be forgotten as your child grown up. With my experience, I realised that it is good to share responsibilities with your spouse because he was also born as a father. I have been lucky to be blessed with the most amazing life partner. We slowly but steady accept our transformation from couple to parent. I decided to make my daughter strong not just mentally but also physically. I have grown up with my daughter and I am still growing up as a mother.

5.

How Life Changes After that first crying!!

If you are a new mom, then welcome to this jolly roller coaster ride. I am a mom of 18 months old beautiful baby girl and life is beautiful. That's one side of the story which covers almost everything (in little). Let's get into the other side of it.

Motherhood is definitely a blessing of almighty. But with this rosy bed, comes the mental exhaustion! Being a first time mom is not an easy job. It is complete transformation of care free woman to caring mom. But you are not alone. Here are some things that I am goes through!

Before I was a Mom... I slept as late as I wanted and lazing it on mornings especially on weekends. I brushed my hair everyday and experiment different hair styles. I and my husband made meals together. I had long gossip on any matter on the phone with my friends and family. I had complete control of my thoughts and my mind. I cleaned my home every day and everything was put perfectly in shelf. I was carrier oriented and always want to be a working woman. I never compromised in any matter. We went for romantic dates. I watched my favourite TV shows regularly without interruption. I loved to read novels in free time. Every month I went for shopping clothes and tried dozens of clothes. I was often travelled alone to my home by bus without thinking the journey was too long. I had never judge myself for taking decisions over meaningless things like buying a chocolates or biscuits. I had never analysed any toddler's poop and piss. I had never washed clothes which are soiled with vomit and poop. I had never gotten up in the middle of the night every hour to check room temperature, night lamp and my location on bed. I had never use mosquito net because I felt suffocation. I didn't know I was capable of feeling so strong. I didn't know the feeling of having my life outside my body. I didn't know that feelings of innocent kisses on my cheeks to realise me how I am important for someone. I didn't know that bond between me and my mom. I didn't know that I could ready to do any sacrifices for someone without any expectations.

But now life is totally changed – I realized that life is not always perfect. And these imperfections are not the end of world. So accept changes and start your new chapter of life as a mother with confidence and be a master in inventing new shortcuts in everything.

I forget my days when I wanted everything perfect. Now quick and easy shortcuts' is a new way to perfection. Here are some things that every new mom like me goes through!

> ➢ I was mentally prepared to stay conscious the whole night for the initial months but to my surprise my girl was a good sleeper in the initial 5 months. But when she was around 6 months old she started waking up more frequently at night. She didn't like to sleep and loved to play at midnight. I tried many ways to increase her sleep time but all my efforts were useless. So I decided to take nap with her at day time and awake at night. I was always feel sleepy and feel that sleep is more satisfying than sex.

> ➢ Now I am able to brush, take shower and get ready in less than ten minutes. She is waiting for me outside bathroom and not given me permission to close the door.

> ➢ I know the detail story of doramon, nobita, motu patlu and all cartoon characters and

only watch these cartoons on TV and now it's difficult to remember my favourite shows.

> I finally understand why my sisters who were mothers of little devils never had time for me to gossip on phone.

> I am easily forget about the hard time she had given me on day time when I saw her sleeping peacefully at night.

> Her dirty diapers are not annoying and I never feel nausea while washing her clothes soiled with pee and poo. (before I felt like vomiting to see my niece's poo and pee. It smells so bad)

> I never prefer to go outside alone but whenever I go I feel incomplete and my mind is constantly thinking about what she is doing right now.

> All her firsts are matter of pride for me. I am always ready to click her all firsts. I also feel

pride even if she gains 100 gm weight. I feel I never love another child as much as mine.

➢ I always dress up her in the prettiest of dresses, click pictures as a professional photographer and whatsapp my family and friends to show off how beautiful my girl is. My face book wall is covered with photos of her first festivals.

➢ After her born, initial 8 months, I started to believe that I am no less than an alien to the outside world. The only regular faces I see is of my husband's (that too when he is back from work and on weekends), my maid and my little girl.

➢ Whenever we went for outing, I packed everything she could possibly need especially diapers but forget my own inner wears.

- She is fond of music and dancing and I jumped with joy when I saw her first moves on the beats of 'Dabang'.

- The bond my husband share with our little angel is so beautiful. Whenever I see him playing with her, I remember my childhood days and miss my papa.

- I never feel awkward to chat with strangers moms who have a small kid and we discussed like expert paediatrician.

- Sometimes I feel wonder how other stay-at-home-mom and working mom deal easily with their colicky and fiercely toddlers.

- When she turned one, I pat myself for the incredible job. And there was a grand celebration.

- I feel so blessed to have a child when I see other couples struggling to get pregnant.

- I understand my real value and strength during this time of my life...I am so usual in getting things done all at once that might surprise my family and definitely my in laws (who always believed I am not able to raise kid and do all other chores without help of them) but the important thing is before I was a Mom... I was never this Happy!

My Life changes 180 degrees after my daughter's birth but the twists and turns taught me many lessons, give me memories and made me peaceful and mature woman. A bond is so blissful, I had never known. Now I am ready be a mom with more passion and confidence.

6.

The first blessing after being mom- breastfeeding

When I was pregnant, I read so much about breast feeding and functions of hormones. My elder sister told me if you plan to breast feed your baby, plan it during pregnancy because after 34 weeks, breasts generally get harder and nipples would not be elastic like before. So I was totally prepared for that and confident to give birth to baby and of course, I did it, successfully! But it is not the end of roller coaster ride. Main task is still remaining.

The hardest challenge was waiting for me and that was Breastfeeding. Breastfeeding is almighty's biggest magic. It's a magical thing that you are able to survive another human with what your body produces! During pregnancy, I thought that Breastfeeding is the easiest and delightful thing to do. But not too late, I understood that the real challenge begins now. Every person I met after delivery asked me only one thing, are you able to breast feed? How much milk I produced? (At that time I felt weather I am buffalo, cow or what) When my daughter was first brought to me for feeding, I had no clues what to do, how to hold her or how to latch her. My mom called nurse. Nurse came in hospital room and just pulled up my gown before I could think or react. My one of the aunt was also came and they all eagerly wanted to check of I am lactating or not! I was in shock that I guarded my body all my life, and here I was, laying naked chest on the hospital bed, nurse and my aunt pumping my breast and a baby trying to latch on! It was painful and depressive experience.

I still remember my struggle in first week the endless hours sitting with breast pump and praying to god for few more drops. Whenever my baby cried because of hunger, I cried too. I was mentally and physically exhausted. My sister gave me advice that I should lock my room so I didn't have any other disturbance, you both feel secure and comfortable and could cuddle her while nursing. It helped in bonding and that further helped in increasing the lactation. I follow her advice and started connecting with my baby slowly which I could not do earlier because of anxiety.

Generally, it may take a few weeks to establishing a feeding schedule for both a new mother and baby to get used to. It is a skill and an important stage for the mother and baby to connect with each other. I realise that breast feeding infants is always at the cost of the mom.

Gradually with the time, me and my girl, learn the method and became comfortable with the entire nursing process. I won the battle when she properly sucked my nipple for the first time and I satisfied her hunger. It was a feeling of completeness. I felt more confident as a mom.

My mom started stuffing me with post-delivery tasteless nutritional food to increase lactation and boost my energy. A good advice given by mom was to try all foods and be sensitive and watchful about what does not suit baby's tummy and moods, follow that pattern and avoid such foods. As a first time mom, I was obviously clueless. But I thankful to my mom and my both sisters who were always there next to me.

The benefits of breastfeeding are known worldwide and government also do lots of campaign. The first yellow drops of your milk is called as colostrums, contains antibodies that protect a newborn against diseases. Besides this it is also rich in proteins that boost infant immunity. There are also lots of benefits of Colostrums that you can surf on internet.

Hence, breastfeeding is the best for your baby. But is it possible for everyone? The reason behind this is 'support'. Breastfeeding is a full time job; it requires your time, stamina, energy and most importantly a strong spirit to continue.

Breastfeeding makes you incredibly hungry and thirsty. Breastfeeding mother needs a lot of care and emotional support. This is the time she needs support from everyone around more than ever. Your spouse is equally responsible for a healthy breastfeeding journey. There were times when I could not even move my body the whole night because my girl was latched whole night and the next morning my body would pain. I lose my temper at times and became cranky. There were days when I feel hungry all time and could not sleep peacefully. I had no time to look into the mirror. Such times, all I expected from my husband was to support me that I'm doing my best. He was also helped me with other household chores and babysitting. It's not easy to be tied up to a tiny human 24×7. I could say, I'm one of the lucky few who had that support and thanks to my family.

Many new mothers are not comfortable with the idea of breastfeeding in public. As a new mom, I was also feeling shame initially. But we had to go for long journey as we lived miles away from our hometown. So with time I understood that it's a natural thing to do. What's the shame in feeding my baby whenever and wherever she feels hungry? No breast could be seen once baby was latched. We as a nation must overcome the childish concept that a women's breast is more of a sexual object than a life giving force. You can't be at home all the time, so sometimes you need to NIP (nursing in public). Breastfeeding is normal process and you should be allowed everywhere because the purpose of all moms is feed the hungry babies.

When she was 16 months old, I was not able to feed her any more. She ate almost everything. Now my breast milk was not enough for her. It was almost negligible. That was difficult for me. It was like giving up full time 24*7 job that had been a part of my life for the last 16 months. I was stay at home mom so every time she wanted to fed, I was there. I feel upset but I knew it had to go but this time passed so quickly. In the end giving up breast feeding taught me that I should not felt insecure. She had her own life and I would be happy with it. Breastfeeding my daughter had been a beautiful journey so far with lots of ups and downs but I had a satisfaction that I did my best that I could do to ensure a healthy life for my girl.

However, many new mothers face challenges during this period of breast feeding. Many new moms not being able to produce enough milk to feed their babies. Family members have to be sensitive towards new mom. Create stress-free environment, give her enough rest, provide her healthy diet and limit her physical exertion. Always trust your body for the milk it makes and love your post-partum body because that has nurtured your little one and most importantly, ask for help whenever you need.

With my experience, I realised problems with breast milk supply are very common but burden of advices given from people are embarrassing for moms who are not able to breast feed. Breast feeding is an extremely important but it does not make you less worthy of being a good mom if you couldn't feed your baby for whatever reason.

Deciding the best way to feed a baby is a very personal choice. It has to be a collective decision of both the partners involved. In bottle feeding, all family members have to share feeding responsibility. For all the new moms, just feed confidently. Motherhood does not only depend on breastfeeding or bottle feeding. So we must support every women's perspective to make the feeding choice weather breastfeed, bottle feed or both because she know and love her child more than rest of the world.

7.

Postpartum blues- you are not alone

Motherhood is definitely a biggest blessing from almighty but it's not at all rosy bed. It is a tiring 24x7 job without leaves. It is both a mental and a physical restless roller coaster ride.

The worst part of motherhood is postpartum blues and no one have the guts to speak about it. This depression is generally experienced by most of the first time mommies but mostly no one prefers to talk about it.

Today I feel proud of the fact that I went through it and came out of it on my own. Today I am going to share with you about my postpartum with lot of confidence.

The main problem is lack of consciousness about postpartum depression among new mothers.

They are afraid to talk about their rainbow of emotions to anyone. When I was pregnant, I read about this on internet but no one ever told me in particular about it. I never thought about it until I experienced it. My family and friends showed me a fascinating picture of my postpartum duration. But no one told me about those silent things that life has thrown to you with child birth. My life is drastically changed after my baby's arrival and I am blissful with this, but at that time it was difficult to understand and accept these changes.

After my daughter's birth, I wanted to be overjoyed and wanted to tell everyone, "Look, I am a mom of cutie pie and I am feeling fantastic." But the joy was still missing. I fought with myself to find out the answers to my questions. However, the more I thought, the more confused I felt. I also felt tired, fussy, boring and sleepy all at the same time. I felt overloaded by this new job as a mother with huge responsibility. I felt that I never live life like free bird as before. Sometimes we need to leave the situation on time. So, I decided to give myself some more time. But I never knew that the days to come will be even more challenging- the never ending feeding, the painful body, the sleepless nights, no personnel life, bunches of laundry, the continuous cries, diaper changing, and negative vibes. And I was in a shock.

Somehow I tried to manage all the things but I was not mentally ready for this. I was not happy and satisfied with myself. I was doing things involuntarily and felt guilty for that. I was afraid to feed her, change her clothes, bathe her, massage her (because nobody was there to help me), I did it anyway because I knew it was my duty as a mom, but all it was to me was a "duty". Still I was not able to fully connect with her. I thought I needed more time to settle myself in this new phase of life. My body was so exhausted due to constant nausea and vomiting during pregnancy and I lost my all positive vibes. I still recall crying like a baby in front of my husband because I could not sleeping for days even after my baby was sleeping peacefully. I was really jealous of my husband because he simply took off for a sound sleep and feeling bad for me that I have to go through all the pain during and after the pregnancy while he was as cool as before. There was so much pressure inside me that everything around me was tedious and every person was giving negative vibes.

The other reason for my depression was the fear that I would never get my life back. I had not known that everything will be fall in pace with time. My family members believe that I am strong and brave girl so they took it for granted that I will understand everything and will easily adjust with the things happening. But this time, it's not true.

Two months passed and gradually things became better (just little bit). And then, one day I got reward for my struggles- the first cute innocent smile. And suddenly I jumped with joy. I smiled back. I clicked lots of pictures and sent to my family and friends. I could accept myself in the new role, but there was a long way to go.

I confess today that I did not fell in love with her the very first time I saw her. I was ambitious and independent girl so constant fear of losing my freedom and identity was pushing me into a depression. And I couldn't even say that to anyone. I was afraid to share my emotions with anyone as I thought that there might be people thinking, that being a mother, you have to be scarifies everything. You have to be responsible and selfless. I was very sure that there was no one who will understand what chaos was going inside me. I never wanted motherhood to be a burden for me. I always wanted to have a peaceful and cheerful motherhood where I look after my baby as well as spend time for myself to achieve my goals.

Time moved on and gradually my depression faded away. Then, one day she called me 'meemee' (means mummy) and there was a spark of joy inside me. I loved the way she was trying to speak and I loved to talk with her in alien language. I loved to watch her innocent activities. I loved to watch cartoons with her. She became my life. I felt loved and responsible too. And of course, I felt finally connected. The gift for me as a mom keep coming in the form of kisses and hugs on fatty belly. I love her all notorious activities. She loved me the most. Her presence encouraged me. In this tough roller coaster ride, I have come a long way. It has not been easy. Motherhood made me laugh, made me cry, made me peaceful, made me love and list went on. And yes, I have loved being a mom. And finally, slowly and steadily the blissful bond has been established.

It went with the endless support from my family, especially my husband. It was him who in reality pulls me out of it. It was his support, patience and encouragement that helped me to come back from depression. He played his role as a father very peacefully and helped me to get my life back. Due to mood swings, I was having difficulty identifying my feelings. Some days I cried for no reason and he sat consoling me. He encouraged me to start writing and work from home. He saved me from many harsh moments of depression. Today I love my daughter more than anything else in the world and she is truly the best thing that ever happened to me. I proudly take her as my responsibility and I am very positive and confident about the way I am raising her. I found that her afternoon nap is 'mee' time and I enjoyed my space. I have started writing while she was napping at afternoon; I am following my dream and also seeing her grow into a beautiful little girl.

She is a happy kid that enjoys outings, being with people, listens to music, singing and dancing.

The main reason behind any kind of depression is we all over-think matters in our life. Due to over thinking, our mind lost the sensation and become numb. It is certainly affecting our life in a negative way. Always remember that you are not sailing in the boat alone. This assurance, that I am not alone helps to pull back you during this phase. The frustration inside is not unjustified. There are many women who have gone through this phase. And today they are happy and confident moms to their children. So for you also, this too shall pass.

One thing that I have realized and I would suggest to all the "would be" and new mums out there is:

-take some time out for yourself. It helps ease your nerves and gives a near aim in life. Always try to get your 'Me Time' from the busy schedule.

-Just remember, your child will observe you. Being happy and portraying a happy mum image in front of your child will create positive vibes in your home and will create a good atmosphere around the child to grow and learn.

-Postpartum depression is the most common outcomes resulting from post pregnancy and no one should shy away from accepting it.

-Have faith in almighty and yourself and be patient, with yourself and the surroundings. Try to be optimist.

- Avoid mental baggage and over stress. Don't expect from others and don't try to meet other's expectations. Never compare yourself with others.

- Letting go of the dream does not mean that we have failed, but simply means that we have created space for new dreams and goals.

- Never re-live in negative memories but hold on to positive memories and reliving them whenever you feel low in spirits.

- Away from negative minded people but spend time only with those whom you can share joy, seek advice from and have fun together.

-We all should feel wonderful about ourselves and very proud of the fact that we have the strength to give birth and nurture a life.

In reality, all the problems are stuck between "matter" and "mind". So, if we don't mind, then it does not matter at all.

8.

How can I forget to be a wife...

One year after my daughter's birth, we had got some time to watch romantic movie while she was sleeping. "It's been a long time when we have seen some romantic movie together", "Will we ever get some quality time or we should try to take out some romantic time for ourselves too??" what you say? My husband asked hopelessly and looks at me as he wanted "our time" in my life. I could sense the disturbance. In reality, it was a long time we had some discussion about ourselves. He simply put his head on my lap and closed his eyes. I observed his face after long time. He looked very tired and lonely. When I moved my fingers in his hair and he slept peacefully, I understood that he was missing his space in my life.

After my daughter's birth, I didn't give much attention on his existence at home and there were assigned tasks lined up for both of us. Our discussion after become parents were restricted only to baby's growth, her food, vaccinations, paediatrician, bill payments and groceries. Whenever we sit together my discussion keeps revolving round my daughter. Whenever we go, I am busy thinking about our little one and then my tired soul want sleep at the end. Sometimes we forget to be a good partner, while trying to be a good parent. After become parents, we could not find the time for each other and became relax. The word "relax" is just a word now without too much value.

Earlier, it was easy when we both were working and living in nuclear set up so we fully enjoyed our space. But then after born of my baby I find it very difficult to comb my hair or take a proper bath. I was more looking like maid then confident working woman. Living in a nuclear setup and raising kid without any support from both set of our parents, we hardly get any quality time for each other. At nights, I was busy in putting baby to sleep and he was still busy in his office work so we were not able to spend good time with each other because lack of time and stamina. I got so busy with my baby or fighting with my own rainbow of emotions that I was giving him negligible time.

For the past 18 months, I totally ignore his feelings because of my hormonal changes, my pregnancy, my mood swings, my delivery, my depression, my little naughty girl ... and what not. My husband always stood as a rock by my side but I did not even notice him as I was busy in my own roller coaster. I want to confess that after become mom, I totally forget to play my role as a wife. All the time I was busy with my baby and household chores. I forgot that he is also just like a kid who needs my time, my attention, my love, my care and pampering. He never complains about it and asks for it. But he loved it when I find a time to sit with him and watch his favourite movie with him.

During pregnancy, he held my hand when I walked with that big baby bump, making snacks for me, satisfying my cravings for sweet at late night and tolerating all the irrational tantrums I threw. We have a healthy child because we both nurtured her in my womb. There might have been times when he might have wanted my time, where he might have wanted to share his feelings with me but I was always busy with this new role as a mom. I want to express regret that even after our daughter's birth when he woke up with me late nights and took care of her, I did not even show gratitude towards him. I was so disturbed about me not getting proper sleep that I forgot that he was also wake up all night and went to work the next morning without even mentioning once what he did. While I could rest a bit with the baby at noon, he could not; still, he cradled the baby in his arms all night so that I could sleep. After become mom, I never asked him about his job, his health and his feelings. I only asked him to help, to do household chores for me, to give him list of things I wanted, to make things easy for me and I can't deny that he did everything. We were just living together under one roof and doing our duties. A "loving Couple" got lost somewhere. Living under the same roof just as parents is not what a good relationship is. He played both the role of a father and a husband but I could not. I forgot that I used to make cards for him; I forgot that I used to give surprises to him; I forgot that I used to make his favourite foods. He loves these small little gestures of mine. After become mom, I neglected him unintentionally and he still love me, he still understand me. I realised effort was lacking from my end. Then I promise to myself that I will try to strike a balance between two roles and I won't irritate him as much as the last two years.

I understood that even after children romance is needed to keep the relationship going. No one wants a relationship where there is no care, love and warmth. To keep the spark of our relationship alive, we can't go for any spa together or I can't think of candle light dinner, no fancy things I can imagine as with our daughter. But other than these I can think of lots of other stuff to ignite our romance.

We decide to keep the phone away and turn the TV off on weekends and holidays. The time we waste in phone or TV we can spend with each other and that would be more valuable. We start to complement each other about our work, giving hugs, hold hands while talking, giving flying kisses if my daughter is present and she also loves to copy it and that means a lot. It's bliss if our kids follow our instruction and sleep early because it gives ample time to parents to spend their special time together. We set up home theatre in our living room using projector is more comfortable and cheaper than go to theatre with our little munchkin. When my daughter gets sleep, we watch movie at late nights. We often dress up and go out for dinner date with our little lady for some change. I started to give him Surprise gifts. No expensive gifts or outing needed. Sometimes I decorate bedroom with red heart shape balloons, make his favourite food, plan to watch his favourite movie, give him a small chit with few loving lines or a small gift or anything small but sweet is enough to bring a wide smile. We plan to cook a dinner together during weekends and trust me it's really fun. We also involve our little master chef. We used to talk about our honeymoon and old good memories that gave us refreshment. We also keep talking about our relationship too, like how it all started and where we are standing now. Whenever get time we are watching our old photos, discuss about our future goals and aims, go to the spot where we first met and so on. This keeps us closer and can help us maintain gracious relation.

So, Lots of effort, energy and time are actually needed to keep the romance alive after kids. So try to balance things smartly and let's give our spouse some attention, time and priority. Loving and caring relationship with our spouse is as important as sleepless nights and screaming baby to keep things going perfectly. Small talks, hugs, flying kisses can go well on daily life without so much effort. So let's try having a strong and romantic marriage keeping all these points in mind.

9.

What   Motherhood   Taught   Me!

Motherhood is a very exploratory thing. You are always trying to do something different that nobody has ever known how to do well. Being a mom is one of the most fruitful and amazing experience of our life but it's not at all easy.

9th November 2015, I delivered baby successfully. When I saw her little tiny innocent face, I started thinking of how she had started to live life independently. She was breathing independently soon after she was born. She had an independent life after nurse cut the umbilical cord. She was no more a part of me physically but of course she was otherwise. But the physical connection had been broken. An umbilical cord raises a baby in the womb until it is ready to get out of the womb into the new world. God created such a magical thing in the form of the umbilical cord through which the mother and the baby share the same bond of feelings.

The umbilical cord is the first toy to each of us. It was also our first mate, supporter and protector. Motherhood has made me wonder about this beautiful creation of love and how all of a sudden the life living inside you, is now outside and visible to you. After birth, the baby is scared to take breaths and feed on its own, learning new ways and techniques. I slowly start to look after and feed her. And then, one day I will have to let go her so the life I have been shielding, takes a flight. An inner clash arises within me. I think of all that I have done for her that was a part of me sometime back. But then, I have to let her go for her own destiny waiting for her. The umbilical cord cut off and your baby taking on its own life into the world is the most satisfied moment for every mother. One cannot hold anything permanently in this world and umbilical cord taught this to us. We always remember that we as mothers are simple care providers. Only a mother understands and feels what the baby feels right from the very beginning when life makes an existence and only a mother knows when to let go too. We simply are made to look after and nourish our child and must do this the best way we can; without expectation of anything. I have given birth to a child, but once she is out of the womb, she is free from me. First she depended for everything on me when she was in womb but slowly she learns to be independent. I have to be cheerful because she is grown up. Then finally one day she will fly away. I as a mom only have to bless her and give freedom her to find her own life and destiny. One thing is definite that your child is not here to fulfil your incomplete dreams and goals. The child is here with his own destiny and he will unfold his own destiny. You can only try to mature and grow yourself. Always remember that how our first connection through umbilical cord becomes our first separation to start baby's new life.

The good thing is that I have never felt that I have made any sacrifices for my child. Because when you feel to do sacrifice for your child, you tend to let the child feel the stress of "I did this for you". I know all about pregnancy, mood swings, the long sleepless nights, postpartum blues and not having a personnel life once a child is born but I believe the decision taken to have a child is because "WE" wish to be a parent. All happiness comes with a price tag but never ever do we want our child to think that we made sacrifices for her. I think it's important that we should change our point of view and do away with the thinking that we are sacrificing everything for our children and they need to be appreciating us. Only a cheerful, positive and satisfied parent can raise a happy and confident child. You do not need to make sacrifices for your child. I am and I will love my daughter more than anyone else will…And I will still be there for her whenever and however she needs me. I am ambitious and carrier oriented woman but I left my job to take care of her but that is my choice... You do not need to use "sacrifice" term as an element so liberally. Do make a choice, but not a sacrifice. So try to be a peaceful, happy and satisfied parent to keep all this points in mind…

10.

Finally, always Love yourself...

I married at the age of 22. I was always a very independent, carrier oriented and ambitious girl. Marriage did not change this part of my personality. After marriage, we were so busy in jobs and fulfil our dreams. We were living in nuclear set up due to job demand and enjoyed each and every moment in life, by giving enough time to each other without disturbance of anyone...Life was perfect, joyful and carefree.

After three years of marriage, we blessed with little angle and then my whole life revolved around her. Waking up at 7am, brush, bath, cook, clean, get ready, nappy changing, feeding, managing home and online business, check facebook, whatsapp and online news, read some blogs, go to market, make rotis, have dinner with husband while my girl was busy in playing with food and made home messy, made an failed attempt to feed her properly, cleaned the kitchen and didn't sleep properly. And alas..! One day, I got exhausted; I realised my life suddenly was moving at an unsounded speed which somehow I was unable to speed up with it. I was so busy in my tedious routine that my personal life ceased to exist. I sat on sofa and thought about what was wrong with me. I had everything with the best amenities at my doorway, beautiful daughter, handsome and loving husband and I still wasn't satisfied. I saw that my husband had maintained his life as cool as before while I over the year had lost my identity because babysitting and household chores became my priority. Is it wrong? No it is not, but what forgetting myself is wrong. Generally, we become so busy to play our role perfect as mothers, wives, daughter in laws forget that before all this we are an individual, an individual who has an identity of her own. I don't want to blame anyone but it's our fault that in this process of progression we had lost a part of ourselves. Marriage and motherhood was never meant to pinch our identity and frankly they did not. We over react when the child is sick, when food is not ready on time or we miss some household chores. In the competition of being the perfect mom and wife, somehow we stop living our lives and start living for others and trust me, I have realised that somehow it is taken for granted that it is our responsibility to manage all. We raise their expectations much higher than our capabilities. I am not talking about a working mom or a stay at home mom but I am talking about the real you.

Tell me one thing: How many of us truly love ourselves like the famous dialogue "main apni favourite hoon" from the one of the bollywood movie. How many of us take out time to pay attention to the needs of our body and mind. We generally take some stupid selfies from an attractive location and update fake status on facebook or whatsapp to show off the world that how much happy we are and love our life. It's not essential to take out time and sit in one corner at home and think over what's happening or what's going to happen. The minute you find happiness in daily happenings, each minute becomes meaningful. In reality, nothing seems to work the way we want. Our life is not fully in our control. The more we try to control, the more stressful we become. We are in some cat race and don't even know about it. Motherhood is not a competition. Don't compare your life with others but try to learn from your mistakes. Always try to be stay fit and healthy. Not only focus on losing weight but also work to build up your stamina, cherish yourself and regain your lost identity.

Being a perfectionist is not a birth mark, its need to be earned but sometimes it's good to be imperfect. We need perfection for inner enjoyment, pleasure and not to show off and definitely not to criticize as well. Sometimes it's good to see things spread here and there, pending work, messy home, uncombed hair, screaming baby. If we break the word Imperfect than it says I m perfect.

So I decided to revisit my earlier life and start enjoying things I used to cherish before become mom. Every morning, just hug myself and start my day with positive affirmations. I decided to contact my old friends, cuddle myself for what I am and stop criticising myself. My personal experience has taught me that becoming a mom is no doubt a life changing event and it changes priorities of life but that does not mean we kill our ambitions and put a full stop on our dreams and live only for our kids. Obviously, I love my daughter most, but I also care for and love myself. Every woman should have hobby to chill out. Marriage and family are important, but so are you! Don't wait for anything to change outside but feel the moment and love your life. Loving yourself first is not being selfish it is just being fair to you. Try to indulge yourself. Take care of your health and happiness. In loving yourself, trust me you are helping those around you, because you will be happier and in turn they would too. It is alright to put yourself first, ok to say 'no'. Be kind to yourself, it is important.

I am in no doubt you all must have read many blogs, articles and heard a lot about love your life and yourself but how much have we implied on ourselves...! We all know life is not perfect and it will never be ....So why not live in a moment and enjoy the imperfection. It works wonders… Celebrate life! Celebrate womanhood!

And always remember that, "The best thing about you is you."

www.ingramcontent.com/pod-product-compliance
Lightning Source LLC
Chambersburg PA
CBHW060757260726
48660CB00002B/659

9 781980 455936